ERECTILE DYSFUNCTION

SURPRISING REASONS FOR ERECTILE DYSFUNCTION

Dr. Andrew Robert

Table of Contents

CHAPTER ONE

ERECTILE DYSFUNCTION (ED)

Erectile issues aren't uncommon - most men experience problems with getting and maintaining an erection now and then. If the troubles persist you may be tormented by erectile dysfunction.

When you get an erection, the blood within your penis will increase. If for any motive the blood glide is limited, your penis will no longer get erect. This will have numerous reasons, from tiredness and strain to an underlying fitness trouble. Up to half of all men aged between 40 and 70 suffer from erectile disorder.

ERECTILE DISORDER PILLS

There are numerous erectile disorder medicines which allow you to triumph over ED and assist you get an erection. All ED tablets currently certified inside the UK basically paintings in the equal manner.

Viagra, Cialis and Levitra all paintings by growing the drift of blood into the penis and they handiest work if you are sexually aroused.

These medications are prescription-only tablets and you need to seek advice from a doctor earlier than you take any of them. You can either go to your GP or use our short and smooth online evaluation. Our on line health practitioner will overview your fitness facts and approve the treatment which is proper for you.

CAN YOU CURE ED?

Whether it's far possible to remedy erectile disorder depends on why you're experiencing troubles. If the cause is an underlying problem which include high blood strain, treating this will most probable enhance your symptoms. If you are experiencing problems due to pressure or tension, lowering the quantity of stress you're underneath could remedy your erectile disorder.

However, for some guys, erectile troubles may additionally persist and represent a everlasting undertaking. This is much more likely to be the case if you are over 60. Erectile dysfunction capsules assist you to manipulate your condition and prevent it from affecting your relationships.

CHAPTER TWO

ABOUT VIAGRA

Viagra may be used as often as as soon as a day each day and generally works inside thirty minutes. The results ultimate for approximately four hours. Viagra is the most well-known and famous of the erectile dysfunction medicines. It includes the energetic component sildenafil, which is likewise available as unbranded sildenafiltablets and over-the-counter Viagra Connect.

ABOUT CIALIS

Cialis generally works in fifteen to thirty minutes, so it's far slightly faster than Viagra and Levitra. The results of Cialis additionally remaining longer – as much as thirty six hours - which make this a popular preference for lots men.

At a low dose of 5mg, Cialis may be taken every day. Cialis each day 5mg is suitable for guys who have taken Cialis earlier than and who've intercourse more than two times per week.

ABOUT LEVITRA

Like Viagra, Levitra normally works inside simply over half an hour. The outcomes closing for about 5 hours (an hour longer than Viagra). Levitra has been in particular shown to be effective in men with diabetes, even though this doesn't imply that Viagra and Cialis will now not work for guys with diabetes.

ABOUT SPEDRA

Spedra works within the identical way as different erectile dysfunction drugs and contains a comparable lively factor. Spedra contains avanafil, which increases blood flow to the penis and widens your blood vessels. It takes impact within 1/2 an hour.

SYMPTOMS OF ERECTILE DYSFUNCTION

The symptoms of erectile disorder are characterised by way of regularly not being able to get or maintain a firm enough erection to have intercourse. Failing to get an erection now and again (for instance, due to drinking an excessive amount of alcohol), or much less than once every 5 instances, is typically not taken into consideration to be erectile disorder. Erectile dysfunction, occasionally called ED or impotence, is very commonplace.

Just under seventy percent of men elderly over 70, and thirty to fifty percentage of men aged among 40 and 70, will enjoy it as a minimum as soon as of their lifestyles. Sadly, it's miles predicted that only 1 / 4 of all men experiencing erectile disorder are searching for treatment.

Often, erectile disorder is a symptom of more serious health problems, so your medical doctor might want to do similarly check to discover the reason of your ED.

CHAPTER THREE

CAUSES OF ERECTILE DYSFUNCTION

Causes of erectile disorder include heart and blood movement conditions such as high blood strain, excessive cholesterol, diabetes, obesity, melancholy, or from a way of life that capabilities things like smoking, ingesting, capsules, overwork, stress, or anxiety. Often the reason is each mental and physical.

Erectile dysfunction can also be because of damaged veins and arteries that constrict the blood's float to the penis, due to deposits of waste and deteriorated erectile tissue. Another purpose could be an damage that has broken the nerves within the pelvic location. It is uncommon for ED to be resulting from a lack of male hormones (testosterone).

WHAT YOU CAN DO

While taking an erectile disorder medication will help you enjoy intercourse and fight symptoms of ED, it gained deal with the underlying reasons.

Depending on your present day way of life you may find that you gain from making modifications which includes:

Weight - If you're obese then losing weight can also enhance your general fitness and sexual feature

Alcohol - Alcohol consumption is also recognized to purpose erectile dysfunction, mainly if you drink excessively or often. Cutting down will help you live healthful.

Smoking - Smoking increases the risk of ED and is a common purpose of cardiovascular problems and ED. Quitting smoking can substantially improve your potential to get an erection.

Stress - Is a totally common purpose of erectile dysfunction in otherwise healthy guys. Reducing strain and making sure which you get enough sleep may have a big effect on your sex lifestyles if your ED is because of strain.

Exercise - Exercising frequently reduces pressure and helps maintain a healthful weight and cardiovascular health, which help prevent erectile disorder.

High blood pressure and cholesterol - If you suspect that your ED can be as a result of an underlying hassle such as high cholesterol levels, you need to see a doctor for similarly tests. You have to also attend any regular health test you are provided with.

SIDE CONSEQUENCES CAN INCLUDE

- Headache

- A flushed face

- Stuffiness within the nose

- Heartburn

common treatments for erectile disorder, there are different remedy options inclusive of:

- Injections into the penis

- Vacuum pumps

- Tablets which are inserted into the penis

If the reasons of your erectile disorder are mental, you could benefit from speaking to a therapist.

A guy is taken into consideration to have erectile dysfunction if he often finds it hard getting or keeping a company sufficient erection so one can have sex, or if it interferes with other sexual pastime.

Most guys have now and again experienced some trouble with their penis becoming hard or staying firm. However, erectile disorder (ED) is simplest considered a challenge if pleasant sexual overall performance has been not possible on some of occasions for some time.

Since the invention that the drug sildenafil, or Viagra, affected penile erections, most people have grow to be conscious that ED is a treatable scientific condition.

Men who've a trouble with their sexual performance can be reluctant to speak with their health practitioner, seeing it can be an embarrassing issue.

However, ED is now nicely understood, and there are numerous treatments to be had.

CHAPTER FOUR

FAST RECORDS ON ERECTILE DISORDER

• Erectile dysfunction (ED) is described as chronic issue achieving and preserving an erection enough to have intercourse.

• Causes are generally clinical but can also be psychological.

• Organic reasons are usually the end result of an underlying clinical condition affecting the blood vessels or nerves presenting the penis.

• Numerous prescribed drugs, leisure tablets, alcohol, and smoking, can all reason ED.

CAUSES

Normal erectile function can be laid low with problems with

any of the subsequent systems:

- blood drift

- nerve deliver

- hormones

PHYSICAL CAUSES

Erectile disorder can cause embarrassment.

It is usually worth consulting a physician about persistent erection issues, as it could be because of a serious clinical circumstance.

Whether the reason is easy or severe, a proper diagnosis can assist to address any underlying medical problems and help clear up sexual difficulties.

The following list summarizes a number of the most commonplace physical or natural reasons of ED:

- heart disorder and narrowing of blood vessels

- diabetes

- excessive blood pressure

- excessive ldl cholesterol

- weight problems and metabolic syndrome

- Parkinson's disorder

- multiple sclerosis

- hormonal issues inclusive of thyroid conditions and testosterone deficiency

- structural or anatomical disorder of the penis, together with Peyronie ailment

- smoking, alcoholism, and substance abuse, together with cocaine use

- treatments for prostate sickness

- surgical headaches

- accidents within the pelvic area or spinal wire

- radiation remedy to the pelvic location

Atherosclerosis is a common reason of blood go with the flow issues. Atherosclerosis causes a narrowing or clogging of arteries within the penis, preventing the important blood flow to the penis to supply an erection.

Numerous prescription medications also can motive ED, which include the ones underneath. Anyone taking prescription medicinal drugs should consult their doctor earlier than preventing or converting their medicinal drugs:

- tablets to govern excessive blood stress

- heart medicines consisting of digoxin

- some diuretics

- drugs that act at the relevant worried machine, consisting of a few snoozing tablets and amphetamines

- anxiety remedies

- antidepressants, which include monoamine oxidase inhibitors (MAOIs), selective serotonin reuptake inhibitors (SSRIs), and tricyclic antidepressants

- opioid painkillers

- some most cancers tablets, inclusive of chemotherapeutic marketers

- prostate treatment pills

- anticholinergics

- hormone capsules

- the peptic ulcer medicinal drug cimetidine

Physical reasons account for 90 percentage of ED cases, with mental causes a whole lot much less not unusual.

CHAPTER FIVE

PSYCHOLOGICAL REASONS

In rare instances, a man may additionally usually have had ED and can in no way have done an erection. This is referred to as primary ED, and the motive is almost usually psychological if there's no obvious anatomical deformity or physiological difficulty. Such mental factors can encompass:

- guilt

- fear of intimacy

- melancholy

- excessive anxiety

Most instances of ED are 'secondary.' This method that erectile characteristic has been normal, however will become elaborate. Causes of a new and continual hassle are typically physical.

Less generally, mental elements reason or contribute to ED, with elements starting from treatable intellectual health illnesses to ordinary emotional states that the majority experience at a while.

It is critical to word that there may be overlap between clinical and psychosocial causes. For example, if a man is overweight, blood float changes can have an effect on his capacity to preserve an erection, that is a bodily purpose. However, he may also have low vanity, that may impact erectile feature and is a psychosocial cause.

DOES USING A BICYCLE PURPOSE ED?

Questions stay approximately the outcomes on guys's health of riding a bicycle.

Some research has raised issues that guys who often cycle for long hours ought to have a higher chance of ED, further to different men's fitness troubles together with infertility and prostate most cancers.

The maximum recent study to investigate this determined that there has been no link among driving a motorcycle and ED, however it did find an association between longer hours of biking and the threat of prostate most cancers.

PROSTATE DISORDER AND ED

Prostate most cancers does not motive ED.

However, prostate surgical operation to take away the cancer and radiation remedy to treat prostate most cancers can cause ED.

Treatment of non-cancerous, benign prostate ailment can also cause the situation.

CHAPTER SIX

TREATMENT

The exact information is that there are many treatments for ED, and maximum men will discover a answer that works for them. Treatments include:

DRUG TREATMENTS

Men can take a set of medicine called PDE-five (phosphodiesterase-5) inhibitors.

Most of those tablets are taken 30 to 60 mins before sex - the best regarded being the blue-coloured tablet sildenafil (Viagra). Other options are:

• vardenafil (Levitra)

• tadalafil (taken as a once-every day tablet called Cialis)

• avanafil (Stendra)

PDE-five inhibitors are most effective available on prescription. A health practitioner will take a look at for heart situations and ask about other medications being taken before prescribing.

Side-results associated with PDE-5 inhibitors include:

- flushing

- visible abnormalities

- listening to loss

- indigestion

- headache

Less typically used drug alternatives encompass prostaglandin E1, that is implemented regionally with the aid of both injecting it into the penis or inserting it down the outlet of the urethra.

Most guys choose a pill, however, so these locally appearing tablets tend to be reserved for guys who cannot take oral treatment.

VACUUM DEVICES

Vacuum erection devices are a mechanical way of producing an erection for men who do no longer want or cannot use drug remedies, or locate they're no longer running.

The penis is made inflexible through the use of a vacuum pump sealed around it that attracts up blood. This is avoided from then leaving the penis by the use of an accompanying band.

The lack of spontaneity with the usage of vacuum devices method that many guys find other remedies for ED optimum.

SURGICAL REMEDIES

There are several surgical remedy options:

• Penile implants: These are a final choice reserved for guys who've no longer had any success with drug treatments and other non-invasive alternatives.

• Vascular surgical operation: Another surgical alternative for some guys is vascular surgical treatment, which attempts to accurate some blood vessel reasons of ED.

Surgery is a closing resort and will most effective be used inside the most excessive cases. Recovery time varies, however achievement prices are high.

Do nutritional supplements and alternative treatments paintings?

The short solution is "no."

No suggestions observed with the aid of docs, nor any established assets of evidence, support the usage of dietary dietary supplements, including herbal capsules.

In addition to there being no evidence in prefer of non-prescription alternatives for ED, the FDA has warned of hidden risks of "remedies" sold on-line.

CHAPTER SEVEN

SYMPTOMS

Men won't constantly effectively achieve an erection, and if this rarely takes place, it is not taken into consideration a scientific trouble.

However, ED does not handiest seek advice from a whole incapability to gain an erect penis. Symptoms also can encompass suffering to maintain an erection for lengthy enough to finish intercourse or an lack of ability to ejaculate.

There are often also emotional signs and symptoms, which include embarrassment, disgrace, tension, and a discounted hobby in sexual sex.

A man is considered to have ED while these signs and symptoms occur regularly.

EXERCISES

There are physical games a man can perform to reduce the consequences of ED.

The pleasant manner to deal with erectile disorder without remedy is by using strengthening the pelvic floor muscular tissues with Kegel exercises. These are frequently associated with women trying to beef up their pelvic place for the duration of being pregnant, but they can be effective for men seeking to regain complete function of the penis.

Firstly, locate the pelvic floor muscle tissues. You can reap this by using preventing mid-move or 3 times the subsequent time you urinate. The muscle tissues you can feel working during this manner are the pelvic ground muscle tissues, and they'll be the focal point of Kegel sporting events.

One Kegel exercise consists of tightening and keeping these muscle groups for 5 seconds after which releasing them. Try to do between 10 and 20 repetitions each day. This may not be feasible while you first start doing the sporting events. However, they have to end up easier through the years.

You need to be able to notice an improvement after 6 weeks.

Make certain you're respiratory obviously at some stage in this technique and avoid pushing down as if you are forcing urination. Instead, carry the muscle groups together in a squeezing movement.

Aerobic exercising, any such jog or maybe a brisk walk can also help the blood to flow into higher and may help enhance ED in men who have stream troubles.

CHAPTER EIGHT

TESTS

The several capability reasons of ED suggest that a health practitioner will generally ask a variety of questions and arrange for blood tests to be completed. Such exams can test for coronary heart troubles, diabetes, and low testosterone, among other things. The medical doctor will even perform a physical examination, together with of the genitals.

Before considering a analysis that calls for remedy, a medical doctor will look for symptoms that have persisted for at the least three months.

Once a clinical records has been installed, a medical doctor will then adopt further research. One simple check, referred to as the 'postage stamp test,' can be helpful in figuring out if the reason is bodily as opposed to psychological.

Men commonly have three to five erections a night time. This check tests for the presence of erections at night time via seeing if postage stamps carried out across the penis before sleep have snapped off overnight. Other tests of nocturnal erection include the Poten test and Snap-Gauge check.

THE END